SEX
CHOCOLATE
CRY

HOW TO STAY HAPPY DURING YOUR MENSTRUAL CYCLE

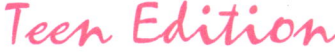

Teen Edition

BY

TAIECE LANIER AND YETUNDE TAIWO

Disclaimer: The examples and stories here are directly related to our personal experiences this is in no way a substitute for a medical experts recommendation. Consult your Physician for medical advice.

DEDICATION

Special thanks to Lanai, a 16 year old senior at Alonzo & Tracy Mourning Senior High Biscayne Bay, Miami, for helping us edit this edition with a teenage perspective. Lanai is Author, Taiece's daughter. She joins us with 5 great years of "AUNT FLOW" experience.

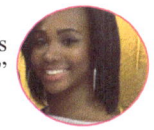

Special thanks also to Ariel, Age 20. She graduated from Monarch High School and is an aspiring Creative Director and Model. Ariel is also the daughter of Author, Taiece Lanier. She joins us with 8 great years of "AUNT FLOW" experience.

Dedicated to all the women who are suffering from their monthly visits from "AUNT FLOW", and need support getting through those irritated feelings, sweet cravings, unexpected boo-hoo moments, cramps, bloating, back pains, eating everything in sight, wishing someone would mess with you just so you could check them and the craving for sex.

We use our experiences and humor to help us get through our menstrual cycle. ENJOY!

THE INTRODUCTION

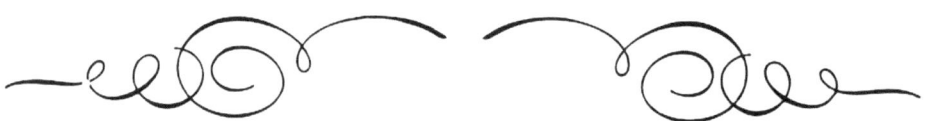

Many men have no compassion for us when it comes to "Aunt FLOW". They cannot understand how after so many years of having the same kind of pain; we are still creating a fuss about it every damn month. Yet, most of them cannot stand seeing us in pain. On average, most girls start their periods at age 12-13.

That means on average, "Aunt FLOW" Will visit you at least 456 times in your womanly lifetime. FUN! WE THINK NOT. Let's step into a humorous way of getting through those few days a month, where life just seems bloated.

Table of Contents

SEX

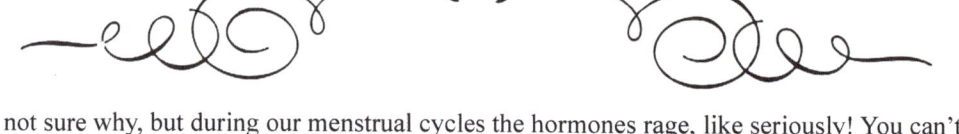

I'm not sure why, but during our menstrual cycles the hormones rage, like seriously! You can't explain what you are feeling and you're feeling extra sensual. DO NOT DO ANYTHING ABOUT. It will pass.

When you're on your last day of your menstrual cycle and you think it's over, Watch "Aunt FLOW" pop up 10 minutes later. Like are you kidding me?

The worst 5 days of my life. Here comes "Aunt FLOW" your hormones are telling you one thing, your mind is reminding you that SEX is not the cure.

Day 1: I'm dying! NO SEX

Day 2: Leave me alone! NO SEX

Day 3: Can we Cuddle! NO SEX

Day 4: I need sweets! NO SEX

Day 5: 24 more hours left ugh! NO SEX

Peer problems. Being simultaneously aroused and disgusted by your own anatomy at the same time. Breath, it's just "Aunt FLOW" she'll pass... Until next month ugh!

Your boyfriend has been pressuring you to have sex. " Wrong time honey, I feel fat, I am insecure, my belly looks deformed and I don't like you right now. Step back" "Aunt FLOW" is in town. Geez!

Having to bring your backpack while going to the bathroom and awkwardly trying to steak-out before the teacher sees you and asks you "why are you bringing your backpack?". In your mind you're like "Are you serious Mrs. Johnson? This is so embarrassing" "ehm, I need to go pee". "Aunt FLOW" problems.

You want to kiss him and yell at him at the same time. Oh! The conundrum.

Don't get hung up on your period. If you were an acrobat before don't stop now! Moving and exercises will actually help you feel better.

Your breasts get plump, and that bra just looks extra sexy and all of a sudden, more boys say hi to you or look at you because you look different. Meanwhile, you feel like crap and probably want to snap their heads off for even looking at you.

You will find that your desire for the opposite sex is heightened. Do not be alarmed if the visions of fantasizing about your crush pops up. It means nothing. I repeat, it means nothing. DO NOT CALL HIM.

2

CHOCOLATE

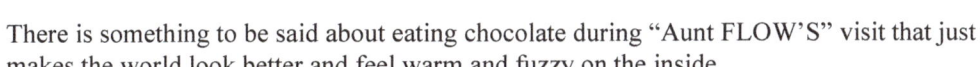

There is something to be said about eating chocolate during "Aunt FLOW'S" visit that just makes the world look better and feel warm and fuzzy on the inside.

I can always tell when my period is coming because I crave nothing but chocolate. Wait, that's always!

How about you sit down to watch TV and you keep breaking that chocolate piece, and then you go to get another piece and realize you ran through that full Hershey's bar in less than 10 Seconds. Feel guilty much! Yah, guilt can suck it! That tasted scrumptious.

My first day is always the worst day, rolled up in my bed, fetal position, heating pad, hair in a high bun and indulging in Godiva covered chocolate strawberries to ease the pain.

If I could chow down spoons of sugar, I would but that's actually bad for you, so I eat some pink grapefruit and baptize it with sugar, then I don't feel so bad.

While I stuff my face with sweets, all I think about is how skinny I want to be.

Try taking a drive when "Aunt FLOW" is heading into town, you'll find yourself buying everything you crave. They say never go to the grocery store when you are hungry. How about never go shopping when you are hungry and "Aunt FLOW" is headed to town. I once bought chickpeas from a period craving. Are you kidding me? Chickpeas? Why? Just because "Aunt FLOW" may want some. Oh! by the way it's still in the pantry months later.

All I want to do is eat chocolate, sleep, and watch a little TV all day.

My 5 days of agony wouldn't seem so bad if every tampon box was like "oh hey, your period sucks, but here is a 50% off coupon for your next purchase of chocolate."

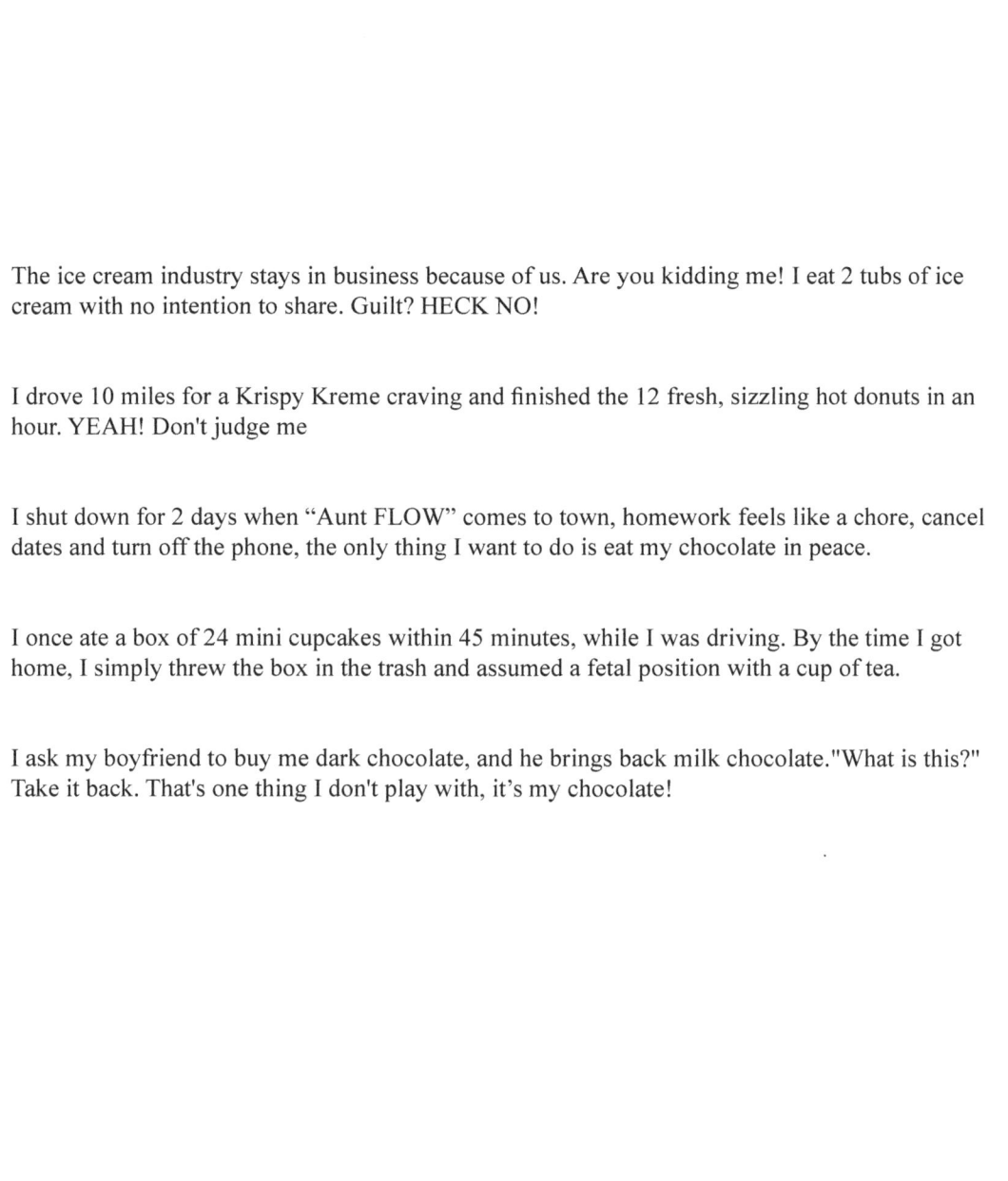

The ice cream industry stays in business because of us. Are you kidding me! I eat 2 tubs of ice cream with no intention to share. Guilt? HECK NO!

I drove 10 miles for a Krispy Kreme craving and finished the 12 fresh, sizzling hot donuts in an hour. YEAH! Don't judge me

I shut down for 2 days when "Aunt FLOW" comes to town, homework feels like a chore, cancel dates and turn off the phone, the only thing I want to do is eat my chocolate in peace.

I once ate a box of 24 mini cupcakes within 45 minutes, while I was driving. By the time I got home, I simply threw the box in the trash and assumed a fetal position with a cup of tea.

I ask my boyfriend to buy me dark chocolate, and he brings back milk chocolate."What is this?" Take it back. That's one thing I don't play with, it's my chocolate!

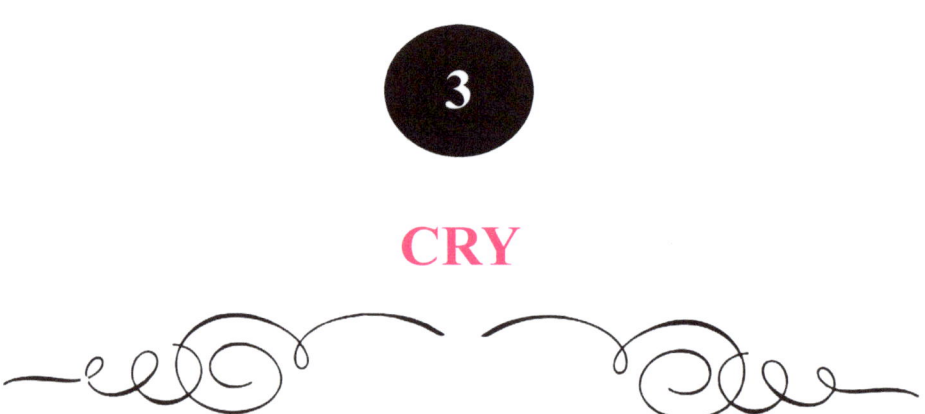

3

CRY

I just feel like crying for no damn reason. Walking around school feeling insecure.

I once cried from getting a hug. I lied and said I was just happy. It was crazy "Aunt FLOW".

I'm in the store and the lady in front of me doesn't have a price on her item, the cashier calls for a price check and I just want to cry! I have my chocolate and Midol in hand and all I want to do is go home! My eyes started tearing up, emotional wreck!

I was driving in my car listening to Mary Mary's 'Shackles' and broke down in tears. I mean boo-hoo ugly cry, so much so, a driver next to me asked if I was okay to which I replied through tears, "I will be okay, thank you." Thanks a lot "Aunt FLOW".

After a few years of "Aunt FLOW", I still don't understand how can my stomach be flat one day and look huge the next. How is this possible. I even have clothes for this time of the month, oh no, not fashionable clothes, but "Aunt FLOW" couture. I wear maxi dresses that are comfortable and allow room for my new figure.

I feel fat, ugly and not sociable during my period. Your girlfriends should understand your desire to be a party pooper and bail frequently.

Don't go shopping on your period nothing you wear is going to look good. Trust me.

Just recently I snapped at a T-mobile phone representative because he sounded rude. I had one of those "I wish you would mess with me" moments. I felt bad, but only after "Aunt FLOW" left.

We feel so powerful and fearless and almost want to dare someone to say something to us, so we can put him or her in CHECK. Ah! I love that fearless feeling. The wrath of a girl on her period. HA!

Crying and looking at yourself in the mirror while giving an ugly cry, and seeing how you look, then crying some more. YES! The release.

That PERIOD headache that it seems even Midol won't help with. My God, who decided this would be a sign for hormone imbalance. Geez "Aunt FLOW".

When your guy doesn't want to see you in pain, in an effort to help, he does this.

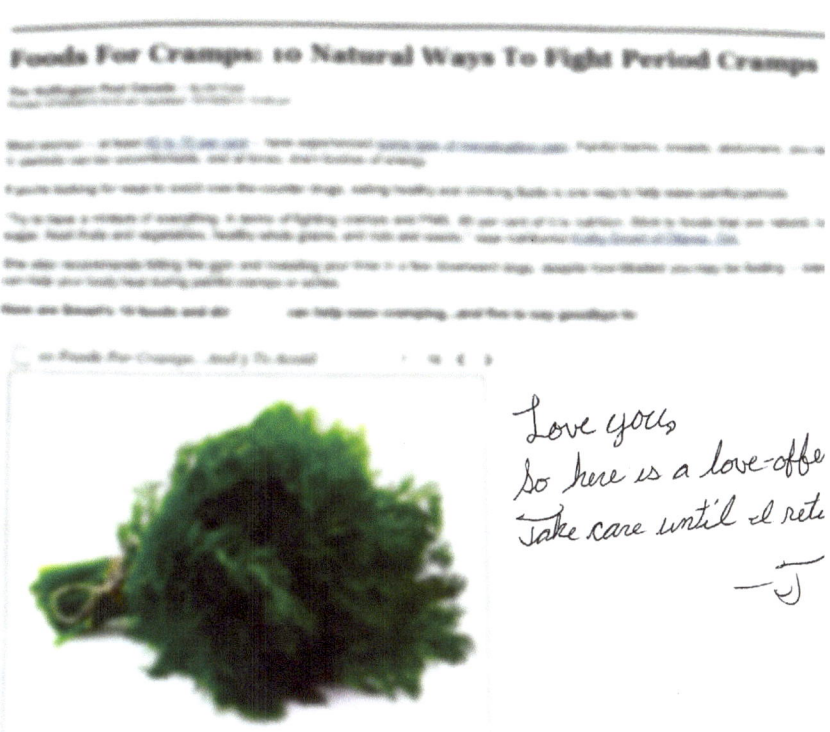

Foods For Cramps: 10 Natural Ways To Fight Period Cramps

Love you,
So here is a love-offe
Take care until I retu

—J

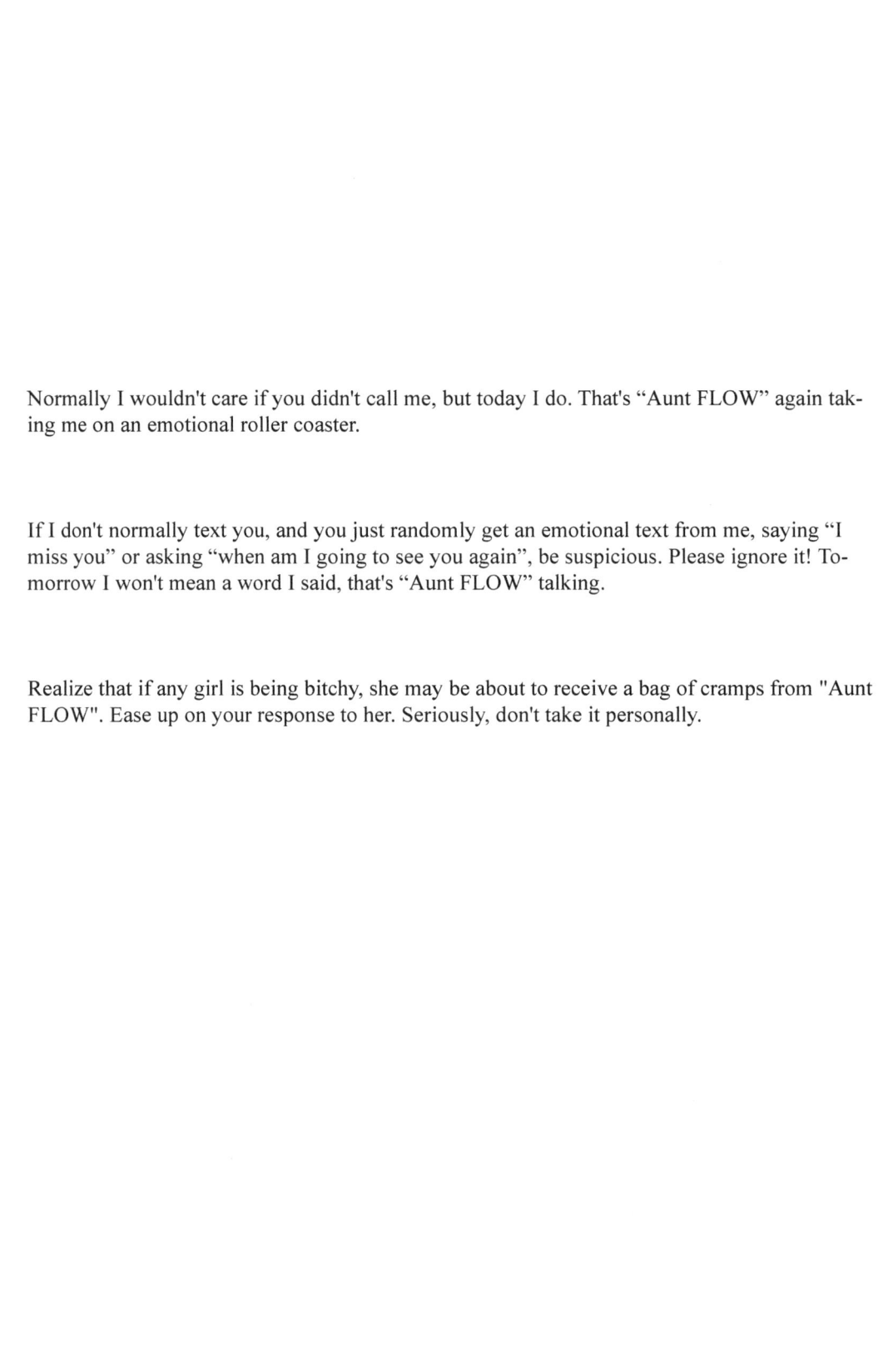

Normally I wouldn't care if you didn't call me, but today I do. That's "Aunt FLOW" again taking me on an emotional roller coaster.

If I don't normally text you, and you just randomly get an emotional text from me, saying "I miss you" or asking "when am I going to see you again", be suspicious. Please ignore it! Tomorrow I won't mean a word I said, that's "Aunt FLOW" talking.

Realize that if any girl is being bitchy, she may be about to receive a bag of cramps from "Aunt FLOW". Ease up on your response to her. Seriously, don't take it personally.

I find that all of a sudden cute little creatures are the most beautiful and most wonderful of God's creations, but if I catch a bug in my house when I am sitting comfy eating my chocolate, while waiting for "Aunt FLOW", Oh! It's going to die, or double die. Then, I cry for killing a living creature. Darn it "Aunt FLOW" ugh!

The irritability is off the scale, my goodness if someone said "hi" to me funny I would analyze what that "sound of hi" really meant. Are you serious? Get out of here with that fatigue "Aunt FLOW".

You feel like opening your brain and pulling out the headache spot then putting it right back.

DO NOT WORRY about the extra weight you gain at that time. Embrace it. It is a part of the cycle, the sooner you get used to it, the better for you.

Hello PPP, YES! Pre and Post Pimples, "Aunt FLOW" wants to make sure the whole world knows she is visiting you, so she gives you loads of dots to sprinkle all over your lovely face. BEAUTIFUL, just BEAUTIFUL.

Why does a pimple show up right on your forehead the night before a big date it's like saying "hey over here", "Aunt FLOW" is coming to town, want to meet her?" *Rolls eyeballs*

You will probably feel like Mother Theresa and feel EVERYTHING. Your empathy for that stray dog or raccoon in your school compound becomes that of a mama goose. GET A HOLD OF YOURSELF PLEASE and remind yourself that "Aunt FLOW" is the cause of this mushiness.

In school, I feel like everyone can see the imaginary period stain on my pants when I'm walking in the hallways. DARN IT "Aunt FLOW"

When you get out of your seat and you feel Niagara falls rush in your underwear.

In school it is normal for you to go up to your girl friends and ask them to " check " you. (for any blood that may have went through your pants) THANKS MUCH "Aunt FLOW"

Waking up to a " murder scene" on your bed from all of the blood that your pad couldn't hold. Really "Aunt FLOW".

For those days when your cramps are unbearable. Maybe I am not on my period, may I am just dying.

Just a heads up ladies. I advice you to make heating pads your best friend.

4

REMEDIES

1. Take Midol as instructed

2. Heating pads can always ease the pain for cramping

3. Force yourself to do some body stretches every morning up to 3 days before your period comes, to help for easier flow

4. Take a warm sit bath, put some Epsom salt for at least 10 minutes a day for the first 2 days.

5. Take a walk and move your body. We know you won't feel like it. DO IT ANYWAY!

6. A cup of warm tea, always sooths the body

7. Get rest, since you are flowing you'll need the energy to recuperate

8. Drink more water than normal, don't worry that you will retain water, you are already bloated anyway, your body needs to stay hydrated, and it will come back to normal.

9. Take Aleve to ease the headache pressure then try to relax your mind and focus on something else, distract your mind

10. Repeat remedies 1 through 9.

AUTHORS

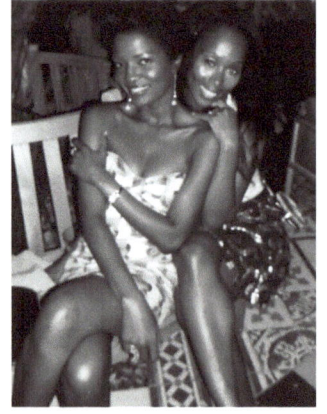

Taiece and Yetunde have been great friends for over 5 years. Their passion for their Businesses/ entrepreneurship and life keeps their friendship growing in Sunny Miami.

This book comes from their love for living life with a side order of humor.
We hope you enjoyed it.

CONNECT WITH TAIECE
www.closeteditors.com
Twitter: @closeteditors
Facebook: Closet Editors Agency
Instagram: Closeteditors

CONNECT WITH YETUNDE
www.icypr.com | www.afropolitanchef.com
Twitter: @yetunde | @afropolitanchef
Facebook: yetunde.taiwo | AfropolitanChef
Instagram: Yetundetaiwo | AfropolitanChef

SPECIAL BONUS OFFER FREE!!! LOG ON TO

www.sexchocolatecry.com/special

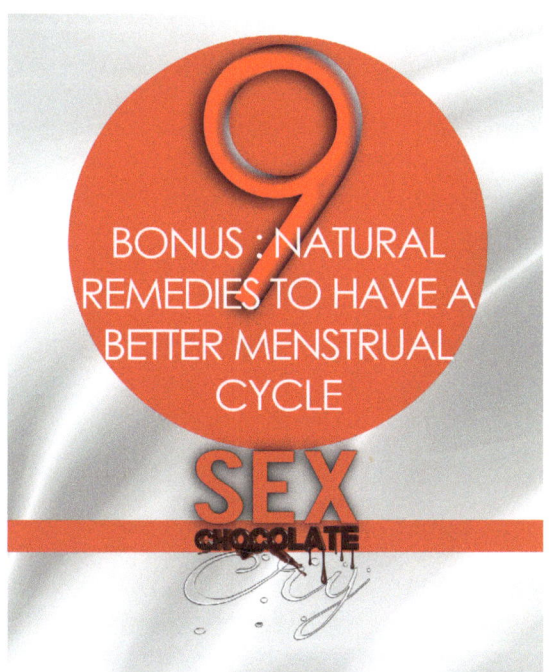

BONUS : NATURAL REMEDIES TO HAVE A BETTER MENSTRUAL CYCLE

Taiece Lanier and Yetunde Taiwo

You and your own Sex Chocolate Cry experience.

***LET US KNOW WHAT YOU THINK ***

So how was that? Bring back any thoughts of your own experience? We hope so, and we hope it made you laugh. When you flip this page, Kindle will give you the chance to rate our book and share your thoughts on Facebook and Twitter. If you believe the book is worth sharing with your girlfriends, please would you take a few seconds to let them know about it? If it turns out to make a difference in their teen, chocolate filled lives, they'll be forever grateful to you, as will we.

For now, appreciate and respect your femininity, eat that chocolate and have a good merry cry. "Aunt FLOW" can't do anything about it.

CONNECT ONLINE: FIND US AT

 WWW.SEXCHOCOLATECRY.COM

FACEBOOK:
 WWW.FACEBOOK.COM/SEXCHOCOLATECRY

TWITTER:
 WWW.TWITTER.COM/SEXCHOCOLATECRY

INSTAGRAM:
 WWW.INSTAGRAM.COM/SEXCHOCOLATECRY

www.ingramcontent.com/pod-product-compliance
Lightning Source LLC
Chambersburg PA
CBHW040329010626
45792CB00024B/2319